SCHIZOPHRENIA

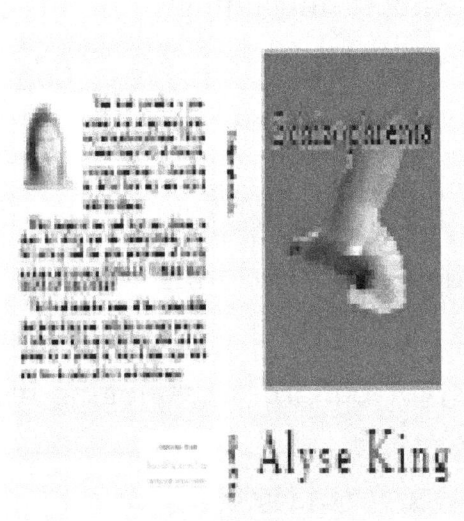

Alyse King

COPYRIGHT

by express, written agreement with the author: Alyse King cmitrainingservices@gmail.com

DEDICATION

I dedicate this book to my beloved son for his strength, courage, endurance and resilience during his most difficult years.

ACKNOWLEDGEMENTS

My deepest gratitude to the Doctors and Nurses, at the Frye Regional Medical Center - South Campus - in Hickory, North Carolina, for their outstanding work in re-evaluating my son's mental illness, and prescribing effective medicines that have paved the way toward his recovery.

Thanks to Larry and Ann who have devoted a tremendous amount of time to help my son overcome this horrific challenge.

Thanks to Trey for his continued friendship and support.

Special thanks to all my dear friends, especially to my dearest friend, Ruth Flowers, who has provided love, friendship and encouragement over the years.

INTRODUCTION

This book provides a panoramic view of my son's journey with schizophrenia. This is a compelling story of strength, courage and hope. It describes in detail how my son coped with this horrible illness.

What inspired me and kept me driven to share his story, was the unforgettable, painful journey and the grim prognosis of nearly no hope of recovery. ... FINALLY, THERE WAS HOPE OF RECOVERY.

This book includes all the coping skills that helped my son with his recovery process. It tells how by keeping his hope alive and not giving up or giving in, helped him cope with over two decades of fears and challenges.

The objective of the book is to increase the awareness of families and caregivers, school counselors and resource officers, psychologist and psychology students. The book gives an overview of how to recognize some of the emerging warning signs of schizophrenia.

The reader has an advantaged point of view as this mother takes you through a journey of hopelessness to the joyous moment that begins the recovery process. This book is intended to assure other families that there is hope of recovery. It includes all the coping skills that helped my son recover from severe paranoid schizophrenia. By maintaining my hope, I helped my son embark on his road to recovery.

The book opens with recounting events of a tragic beginning that ended with receiving proper medical care. It contains a detailed description of my son's schizophrenia from a mother. The second section focuses on the coping process, the hope, the endurance, the strength and the resiliency. The final chapter discusses the dramatic recovery process of my son.

May this book console you because YES, there is life after learning how to cope with paranoid schizophrenia.

HOW THIS JOURNEY BEGAN

It was April 1991, and another beautiful spring evening in Southern California was coming to its close. That beautiful day would turn into the worst day of my life. Unexpectedly, I was about to embark on a long, heart-breaking journey into the unknown that would forever change my life.

It was now a little past midnight. I was sleeping in my downstairs bedroom. My four children, three daughters and one son were all asleep in their rooms upstairs. That night, when my son came into my room, and sat on the edge of my bed, I was fast asleep. As soon as I saw him, I immediately got up and I knew something was wrong.

I got up as quickly as I could and sat next to him because I could clearly see he was in distress. At first, he was quiet, but distracted. I started to panic, but I tried hard to stay calm. I realized that my greatest fears were coming true.

While I reached out and held his hand, I asked him what was wrong. He was looking very frightened and told me he could not fall asleep. He then said to me, ***"Mom, I don't know what*** *is happening to me, something is wrong. I feel like a baby."* I felt my heart stop beating. I became very distressed. I asked him if he would like to go to the emergency room. I knew I had to do something. I must quickly get him to a doctor. But, of course, like the countless times before, he refused.

I stayed up trying to comfort him the best that I could. I told him that I loved him. I tried to give him hope by telling him he would be ok in the morning. He went back upstairs to his bedroom, and I fell back to sleep. Although for the past couple of years, there were many subtle warning signs that a serious mental breakdown was imminent, I didn't realize that, on this night, his life had taken a dramatic turn.

It was now morning and I immediately got out of bed to check on my son. He was still awake, and pacing around in the house. He appeared very disconnected, something was very wrong with him. He was not hearing anything that I was saying. He was clearly distracted. I knew that he needed urgent medical attention. I became very nervous.

Again, I tried to take him to the hospital, but I could not convince him to go. He resisted my attempts to maneuver him into my car. At that time, the thought of dialing 911 did not occur to me. I simply kept comforting him. Later in time, I realized that I had made a serious mistake by not dialing 911.

I made one of the greatest mistakes of my life!

Instead of dialing 911 for help, I foolishly went to work that morning to ask for time off to take care of my son. At that time, I was very much afraid of losing my job because I was the sole provider. I had no idea that a drama was unfolding and the worst was yet to come.

Before I left for work that morning, I called one of my friends, and told her what had happened the night before and that morning. She suggested that I immediately take my son to the doctor.

I then made the greatest mistake of my life! Perhaps, it was out of sheer ignorance or simply just panic. I made my son a cup of hot mint tea and told him that I would return home within two hours. I left him sitting at the dining table with the cup of tea, and went to work.

One may ask, **"How could I make such a foolish decision?"**

The answer is *"I was afraid of losing my job."*

As it turned out, my boss was not in that day.

That situation turned out to be the worst decision I had ever made; one that I would regret for the rest of my life.

While at the office, I received a phone call from my friend with whom I spoke earlier that morning. She told me that my son had called her several times that morning, and that those calls disturbed her very much. I told her that I was leaving work to take him to the hospital.

My friend said she had supplements at her house that would help my son and that I should stop by and get them.

I immediately left the office and drove to her house. When I arrived, my son was talking to her on the speakerphone. I heard a little of the conversation and it scared me so badly that I was paralyzed. My friend told me to return home as quickly as I could.

I ran, jumped into my car and drove home as fast as I could. As I got out of my car and walked to the front door on that beautiful spring morning, I felt an air of eeriness. **Something was going wrong in my house. I could sense it. I could feel it.**

Before I left for work that morning, I remember opening the curtains. However, when I returned home, the curtains were closed.

As I opened the front door and stepped inside the house, my heart raced. My son did not acknowledge that I was there; it was as if no one had entered the house. I was terrified, and for good reason. Grave danger loomed. I must act quickly.

One can only imagine the heart wrenching feeling I had at this time.

My son was in extreme emotional agony and pain and in desperate need of help. He was paranoid and delusional. He kept talking to himself, pacing around the house, and could not stop. The cup of tea I had made him earlier that morning was still on the table, untouched. All that was on my mind was getting him to the hospital. His behavior was strange, something

I had never seen before. I kept comforting him because that was necessary for his survival. I kept reassuring him I loved him and that I am home to stay with him. I told him that everything would be ok, that we just needed to get to the doctor. He continued to be distracted and unresponsive. He had no joy, no emotions; he was disorganized and disconnected.

He continued relentlessly pacing back and forth. I tried to comfort him because it was clear to see that he was in anguish and much distress. Nothing I tried was working. As I was communicating with him, he would not give me a clear response.

I tried to get him into the car to take him to the hospital but he kept refusing. Everything I tried failed; I was very unsuccessful. He continued talking with all disconnected sentences, nothing was making sense; he was completely incoherent.

I kept trying to comfort him, but the truth was that I was very frightened and uncontrollably shaking. I wanted to take away his pain and suffering. He had a look of desperation in his eyes, as if asking for my help. I desperately kept trying to get him into the car. I could not get him into the car. Of course, it was impossible for me to get him to the hospital given his broken mental state. His condition was grave and I was powerless.

Still, I did not dial 911. To this day, I cannot explain to anyone why I did not pick up the telephone and dial 911 for help. Maybe I was waiting for a miracle. **I JUST DO NOT KNOW.** I remember that I kept trying to comfort him, and kept telling him everything would be ok, but that promise turned out to be false.

As I tried to think what next to do, my son briefly sat down at the dining table and I sat down with him. Suddenly, he jumped up from the chair, and to my shocking surprise, he leaped over the table, went into the kitchen, and took a large kitchen knife out of the drawer. He then turned sharply towards me and in a weird voice shouted, *"DON'T MOVE."* It startled me.

A great fear overpowered me, and it was paralyzing. *"Was I going to die?" "Are we both going to die?"* I immediately dismissed that thought.

I was scared to death of what might happen. I tried hard not to show my fears because I did not want to startle him. I then begged him to put down the knife. He could not reason, and talking to him was not working.

"What am I going to do to get out of this alive?"

I started to pray.

I remembered how much I was trembling with fear, but remained stoic. I did not want my son to see that I was deathly afraid of that kitchen knife, and I kept thinking about how terrifying he must be feeling.

I kept wishing that this were a terrifying nightmare. Only this was not a usual nightmare. This was a real life, wide-awake nightmare.

Still trembling, I slowly and carefully moved toward him. I kept talking to him with consoling words: *"Son, this is mom; you are going to be ok, give me the knife."* I remember how desperately I tried to get the knife out of his hand and away from him as quickly as I could. But to no avail.

Again, he lifted the knife, pointed it at me and shouted, *"DON'T MOVE."* I stopped. I was motionless. I wanted to reach out to help him, to take him into my arms, to hug him, comfort and reassure him that he would be all right. He would not let me move. This went on and on and on for quite a while.

The telephone was on the dining table next to him. I wanted to reach out and grab it as fast as I could to call for help, but I was motionless. I was afraid of how he might react. I could not take the chance of what my moving might trigger in him. I just could not get to it.
By this time, he had deteriorated into a total psychotic break with reality.

After what appeared to be an eternity, he appeared calm for only a few moments. I gradually moved toward the front door, but before I got there, he shouted at me, ***"STOP."*** I stopped, and slowly backed away. I kept pleading with him to put down the knife.

I tried moving to the back door, and again he stopped me. After several minutes had passed, I again slowly tried moving to the front door, but could not. This time he was more agitated than ever. He shouted again, ***"STOP, DON'T MOVE."***

I knew that my son was more frightened than I could ever be. I kept waiting for an opportunity to escape, to run screaming to anyone who could help me.

I was alone in the house with my son. Earlier that morning, my three daughters left for school. I thought about screaming for help in hopes that someone would hear me, but my neighbors were not home.

With the knife still in his hand, I thought death was imminent for both of us. With the magnitude of symptoms he was experiencing, anything dreadful could happen.

I started to pray aloud and continued praying. That was now my only option. Those words that filled my desperate prayers were my only comfort.

To my greatest surprise, my son began calling aloud to God to save him. In the depths of my deepest sorrows and fears, I was extremely proud of my dear son for his strength and courage. In the midst of having a full-blown psychotic breakdown, my son displayed a courageous act of faith and trusted that God would protect him. "

"Just keep praying," I kept telling him. *"Keep praying. Keep praying. Don't stop, keep*

praying." I remembered repeating this over and over.

We both kept praying aloud, *"Dear God, please help us."* We both kept repeating those word, *"DEAR GOD, please help us."* That went on for a long time. All the while, the knife remained tightly gripped in his hand, and I still could not move.

The clock slowly ticked in the kitchen: *tick, tick, tick*. I nervously waited for help to arrive. It felt like an eternity. *"Where will help come from, and how will it help us?"* I kept wondering, and wondering and wondering and praying and hoping. I held back my tears.

Unexpectedly, the telephone rang. I leaned over to answer it, but he grabbed it from the receiver and said, *"Hello,"* in a strange voice. Next, he said, *"SHE IS NOT HOME."* I remained motionless.

'SHE IS NOT HOME,' echoed through my mind, and I trembled even more than before. *"Was I going to die? Were we both going to die?"*

I could not bear that thought. He then slammed the phone onto the receiver. My heart plummeted. With the knife still in his hand, I feared for our lives more than ever before. I continued praying for help.

What could I do? I needed to do something, but I could not move.

I became convinced that the key to my -- to our -- survival was for me to remain calm and unafraid. I needed to clear my mind. I needed clarity. I had to focus. I had to clear my mind.

After what seemed to be hours had passed, I was happy to hear the phone ring again. I kept thinking, *"I must do something to get help. What can I do?" "Should I make a dash to one of the doors when he answers the phone?" "Should I risk it?"*

He is much faster, bigger and stronger than I am. Should I risk it?

Again, he picked up the phone, and said, *"SHE IS NOT HOME."* The caller said something, and he replied, *"I DON'T' KNOW WHERE SHE IS."*

That moment was one of the worst moments of my life. Trembling with fear, I stood right in front of him. *'I don't believe this is happening,'* I kept thinking.

"Dear God," I prayed again, *"please help us both."* Before he could hang up the phone, I started to scream at the top of my voice, *"I am here. I am here. I am home. He won't let me talk on the phone."*

He quickly put the phone back onto the receiver and shouted at me to be, *"QUIET."* I was **TERRIFIED**! I continued to remain calm, and I kept comforting him because I felt he was more frightened than I was. I was 100% more worried for his health than I was for my safety.

After more time had passed, the telephone rang a third time. *To this day, I do not know if the call was from the same person or if different people were calling.* He answered again, and said, *"SHE IS NOT HOME."* Again, I started screaming at the top of my voice. *"Help me, help me, help me,"* in a more urgent voice. *"He is going to hurt me, he has a knife." "He locked me in the house, and I cannot get out."* I kept repeating that before he hung up the phone.

As his mother, I really did not believe or feel that my son would injure himself or me only because hurting people was not a part of his nature. Sure, I expressed concern because a knife was involved, and because he was hallucinating. I kept busy trying to comfort my son. However, I was consumed with fear.

I kept waiting, and not losing hope. "We must get out of this alive," I kept telling myself.

As time slowly dragged on, my hopes and prayers of getting out of this dire situation began to diminish. Again, I begged God to rescue us. I waited. It seemed that my faith, and trust in my prayers were being tested. However, my prayers would become the cornerstone to us surviving this situation.

My heart began beating faster and faster while his condition was getting worse in front of my eyes.

I needed help and had to do something. Could I tackle him? Could I manage to overpower him? No, we might both die with just one sudden thrust of that knife. How can I get help?

There were many disconnected dialogs between us, many too traumatic for me to re-visit.

As I anxiously waited for rescue, I heard a faint sound that came from the front of the house. Since my son would not allow me to move, I could not look to see what, or who was outside. After a few seconds, there was dead silence.

After a little while, I heard the sound again. This time it was louder than before. As I attempted to move toward the front door to where the sound seemed to have originated, he instantly jumped towards me, and told me not to move. I knew he heard that sound because he turned and looked at the front door. I pleaded with him to let me peek through the curtains to see who was outside. He did not respond. Rather, he kept repeating, ***"Don't move."*** Then total silence, again.

After even more time had passed, we heard the sound a third time; this time it was louder and closer to the house. This time as I tried to move towards the sound, for whatever reason, my son did not stop me. I slowly walked to the door, turned the knob, opened the door and looked outside.

Imagine the scene that I am about to share with you. To my complete surprise, I saw two police officers with guns in their hands, stooping along the side of the neighbor's house directly in front of my house. Both officers gestured to me, and said, *"RUN."* I did not run to them. I walked towards them, begging them to *"Please help my so, he is sick."* The officers kept motioning to me, and kept saying, **"RUN."**

I refused to run to them because I did not want to scare my son. I only wanted to protect him. Even though I was frightened of the knife in his hand, I truly did not believe that my son was going to harm him or me. As I hurriedly walked towards the officers, I turned, looked and saw my son running up the stairs with the telephone in his hand. The officers now pointed their guns directly at the front door as if they were going to shoot him.

I was terribly frightened! I thought they were going to shoot and kill my son. I felt I was going to have a heart attack and started panicking.

I kept praying, *"Dear God please help me again. Please stop them from killing my son."*

Immediately, I began screaming, *"DON'T SHOOT, DON'T SHOOT, DON'T SHOOT. HE'S SICK."* I kept yelling as I grabbed onto the arm of one of the officers, *"Please don't shoot him, please take him to the hospital,"* I kept pleading with the officers.

Within minutes, I saw several more police officers swarming throughout the yard.

After a few minutes, my son was in full psychosis; hallucinating and paranoid. He came out of the house, threw the knife in the grass and walked towards the officers and me. He kept praying, *"Oh God, please help me."* *"Oh God, please help me."*

The police ordered him to put up his arms. With guns still pointed at him, several of the officers surrounded him, handcuffed him and put him into one of the police cars.

Other officers entered the house and began questioning me. I told them everything that led up to that moment and kept pleading with them that my son needed medical care. A few of the officers left the house, and, naturally, I assumed that they were taking him to the hospital.

Two of the police officers remained behind and continued questioning me. They now focused on whether my son was a drug user. I assured them that he was not a drug addict and had never used drugs of any kind.

The police wanted proof that my son was ill. I provided them the information. They called the Psychiatric Clinic to which I had taken my son for treatment, and spoke to the intern psychologist. They spoke to the same person who, two weeks earlier, told me that my son was not ill.

At that time, the intern Psychologist said to me, ***"I know what's wrong, there's a mother-son thing going on."*** I could not believe what I had heard. I thought this person was a nut, an absolute FOOL. My son and I immediately left his office and never returned.

After the police officers left my house, alone and broken hearted, I broke down and wept. After a while, I got up, dried my tears and telephoned the police station to ask to which hospital they had taken my son.

The worst was yet to come.

Imagine how shocked I was. My very sick son was not in a hospital! **THEY LOCKED HIM IN A JAIL CELL!**
HOW TRAUMATIZING IT MUST HAVE BEEN FOR HIM!

The person with whom I spoke at the police station told me they were observing him in jail. ***My son desperately needed medical care in a hospital, NOT IN A JAIL.***

Although I was grateful to the officers for rescuing both of us, they were 100% wrong to jail my son. He was clearly having a psychiatric breakdown. Even an untrained person could clearly recognize that a person in such a state of psychological distress needed to be in an emergency room.

Obviously, from my experience, I do not think those officers were trained to handle crises involving mentally ill individuals, and involuntary commitments. The way in which they handled my son was traumatic.

Finally, after several hours, my son was transported to a psychiatric hospital.

(The decision I made that day to leave my son and go to work turned out to be one of my biggest mistakes; I will regret it for the rest of my life. That decision has haunted me for over two decades. I learned that no matter what the cost, my children's health – NOT A JOB -- should be my first priority.

From the moment he held me hostage with that knife, my choice was clear. I had to accept the overwhelming responsibility of giving up my job to stay at home to care for my son. I didn't work outside my home for the seven long years that I devoted myself to caring for my son.)

A SHOCKING DIAGNOSIS

It would be the third psychiatric hospital that would make a diagnosis that rocked my world. The first two hospitals spared me from the inevitable. I waited for the diagnosis in the psychiatrist's office at the hospital. I was alone, scared, and sobbing.

As I sat grief stricken and weeping in the doctor's office, my mind reflected on the time when my son was a healthy baby boy, who grew up to be a fine 18-year-old young man. He loved life, loved the outdoors, loved sports and loved people. He was sweet, caring and kind to everyone. He was a son any parent would want to have. Now, he is behind cold, scary walls of insanity.

Frightened and alone, I needed comfort. I needed strength. No one was there to comfort me. I dreaded waiting for the psychiatrist, and dreaded the diagnosis even more. I knew it was not going to be good. I silently and repeatedly prayed.

"GOD, PLEASE HEAR MY PRAYERS AGAIN. PLEASE GIVE ME STRENGTH AND WISDOM MORE THAN EVER."

My heart ached and my spirit was low. I wanted to die to spare myself the pain. Minutes passed stretching into what seemed to be hours.

The doctor finally arrived, and sat at his desk. My mind raced to thoughts of hearing good news from the doctor, maybe my son could come home the next day. To my greatest dismay, the situation worsened.

I then heard two words from the doctor, ***"Paranoid Schizophrenia."*** I did not know what those words meant. All that I remember is that those words sounded awful. I dreaded them. I knew paranoid was not good, but I could not recall ever hearing the word schizophrenia. **"SCHIZO WHAT?"** I asked the doctor.

That moment was one of the most agonizing moments of my life.

Schizophrenia had eeriness to it. Alone and trembling, my emotions ran the gamut. First, I was shocked. Then I was numb. Then I was filled with grief and sadness. I felt my chest tighten. I was panicking. I wanted to run upstairs, open those large, locked steel doors, and rush to my son.

I FELT TOTALLY DEFEATED.

I was in agony. **"My son, how can I protect you from this tragedy?"** My eyes filled with tears. As I wept, my only comfort was that my son would finally get the MEDICAL TREATMENT that he desperately needed. All I wanted was for him to recover and return to being the son any parent would want to have.

Only a few floors above, locked behind large doors, pacing aimlessly, incessantly, talking to himself, looking frightened, was my 18-year-old son. *"MOM WHAT IS HAPPENING TO ME? WHAT IS HAPPENING TO ME?"* he repeatedly asked me when I went to see him. I continually tried to comfort him and reassure him that he would be fine.

Nothing in my life could have prepared me, or given me any comfort for this diagnosis. It was a severe blow to my family. I went home and wept until I had no more tears.

THE PROGNOSIS

That day would turn out to be one of the worst days of my life. I was at my lowest point when I heard the words, *"LAW OF THIRDS."* That was my son's prognosis. The psychiatrist explained what that meant but I could not fully comprehend all that he was explaining to me. I began to cry uncontrollably while my mind drifted back to the time when my son was a happy, healthy young boy.

The doctor continued explaining that, *one third of patients will recover and lead normal lives, one-third will stabilize but will not return to normal, and one third will not recover, they will remain ill.*

Was this prognosis hopeful or hopeless?

I knew the magnitude of this illness would be far beyond my comprehension. More than ever, I now needed to rely heavily on my faith and my God to sustain my children and me. I was sure that I could rely on my unfailing love for my children and my faith as they have always strengthened me.

Finally, I could no longer bear it. I asked the doctor, **"WHICH THIRD APPLIED TO MY SON?"**

Before the doctor could reply, I continued with my silent prayers.

"DEAR GOD, PLEASE, LET HIM BE IN THE THIRD THAT RECOVERS."

Of course, I knew now that at that moment there were no answers to that question. Only time would tell.

Not everyone will feel the same emotions that I felt after such a grim diagnosis.

**In my grief, I questioned myself.
How will I handle this?
Will I have the strength?
How will I help my son?
How will I deal with these immense challenges and not become overwhelmed?**

There were more unanswered questions than answers. It was clear that I would now live a life filled with many uncertainties.

Although this was a challenging time in my life, it gave me the opportunity to learn about the causes, effects and treatments of mental illness. When I first learned that my son had a disabling illness that has no hope of a cure, (anytime soon), a torturous death could not have brought more pain. This was the most abysmal period in my life.

As the illness progressed, it was about to take my son's life on an unexpected, cruel and heart wrenching journey. Great challenges lay ahead on this journey. This journey would devastate his life for decades. The choice was clear. I would stay home and care for my son. Sadly, despite my best efforts and with the best medical care available, it was heartbreaking that my son's mental health continued to decline.

From a shocking diagnosis and a disheartening prognosis of practically '**no hope of recovery**,' to glimmers of hope of recovery, then on to the recovering period. This progress has encouraged me to write this book to promote a mentally healthy America one person at a time, one family at a time, one community at a time, one city at a time.

WHAT IS SCHIZOPHRENIA

No matter how schizophrenia is defined, it is impossible to explain the full magnitude of the destructiveness of this illness.

According to the Encarta Dictionary, *"schiz-o— phre-ni-a, is 'a severe psychiatric disorder with symptoms of emotional instability, detachment from reality, and withdrawal into the self.'"*

According to the National Institute of Mental Health (NIMH), *"Schizophrenia is a chronic, severe and disabling brain disorder that has affected people throughout history."* About 1% *of Americans have the disease. Specifically, 1-2 percent of Americans who are 18 and older are affected in any given year. The article goes on to state,* *"Scientists have long known that Schizophrenia runs in families ... it occurs in 10% of people who have first-degree relatives with the disorder."*

According to the World Fellowship for Schizophrenia and Allied Disorders, *"Schizophrenia is the most persistent and disabling of the major mental illnesses...While it is treatable in many cases, there is yet no cure..."*

A Medical Journal, Current. Opin. Psychiatry 16 (2) 2003 contained the quote, *"It is well known that schizophrenia is a chronic, generally life-long, mental illness that significantly debilitates afflicted individuals and severely compromises their function and quality of life."*

The Nutritional Management of Schizophrenia described it in this way, *"Schizophrenia may be caused by genetic predisposing factors or environmental influences."*

University of Alberta Press Release, states, *"Schizophrenia is a biochemical brain disorder characterized by delusions, disordered thinking, hallucinations and a lack of motivation and energy."*

William Carpenter, Director of the Maryland Psychiatric Research Center stated, *"It's a terrible disease and major public health problems."*

Daniel Weinberger of the NIMH stated, *"Whatever the anatomical change in schizophrenia, it's a very small one. This is not a stroke. This is not a massive failure of brain development - this is a subtle, subtle defect."*

According to the World Health Organization, (WHO), Media Centre dated June 2007,

Geneva, *"There are nearly 54 million people around the world with severe mental disorders, such as schizophrenia and bipolar affective disorder (manic depressive illness). In addition, 154 million people suffer from depression."*

National Alliance on Mental Illness. (NAMI) stated, *"Schizophrenia is a serious mental illness that affects 2.4 million American adults over the age of 18."*

Regarding one possible cause of Schizophrenia, the American Psychiatric Association is convinced that, *"Although the origin of Schizophrenia has not been identified, Scientists know that there are...hereditary or genetic predispositions for the disease because it runs in families."*

If these reports are correct, Schizophrenia may strike anyone at any time. It has no barriers, no boundaries no ethnic demarcations and it does not discriminate. It strikes those in every class, in every occupation, the young and old, man and woman, rich and poor, blacks, whites, browns, and all other colors. It strikes the educated and the illiterate, the powerful and the famous as well as movie stars, those with prestige and those who have achieved in every field. It does not discriminate based on religious affiliation, cultural background or economic status.

Since it strikes anyone at any time, it could be: a spouse, a father or mother, a son or daughter, aunts or uncles, nieces or nephews, cousins, friends, neighbors, workmates, school mates, acquaintances or YOU.

It has been said that, 'knowledge is power.' Knowledge saves lives from the bitter effects of mental illness.

In reality, no scientific research has resulted in findings to support a possible cure. Based on this fact, for decades my son's outcome appeared grim. However, thanks to modern, effective and available medicines the intensity and frequency of the illness are manageable. While the illness continues to cause minor impairments in function despite treatments and family support, my family and I successfully live with this illness.

If mental illness is untreated, or if not treated in a timely manner, the frightening reality of suicide is a possibility. The quicker one begins the right treatment program, the better the chance of recovery will be.

The cause of Schizophrenia is still unknown. Fortunately, for the estimated 10% of the American population, and their families as well as friends and communities, who are affected by this illness, many excellent anti-psychotic medications are currently available.

Schizophrenia is a mental illness that causes unusual thinking and feelings. Many people who have this illness experience auditory hallucinations, psychosis and delusions on an ongoing basis.

Psychosis is a *"psychiatric disorder that is marked by delusions, hallucinations, incoherence, and distorted perceptions of reality,"* states the Encyclopedia Britannica.

"Delusions are false beliefs that are not part of the person's culture and do not change. The person believes delusions even after other people prove that the beliefs are not true or logical," states the National Institute of Mental Health (NIMH), March 2012.

WARNING SIGNS I MISSED

Imagine your young child acting a 'little strange', 'weird,' or a 'little odd', bizarre, or 'peculiar.' Perhaps, making a strange comment, a strange sentence or even saying strange words.

This went on for several years, until, I woke up one night and those little odd behaviors were not at all odd, rather, they intensified and turned into a full-blown, paranoid schizophrenic episode. The shock, the horror, the pain, the grief, the disappointments and the regrets were unimaginable.

The anger I felt because I missed those subtle warning signs of mental illness were also unimaginable as was the pain and sadness because I did not help my son, when I could have. But, the worst experience was my horrible feelings when others laughed and joked that my son was weird. Unknowingly those 'odd,' 'strange,' and 'peculiar' behaviors were the symptoms of mental illness. They were signs that only I saw. My son's young life was already derailing. A turbulent life had already begun for my family. Gone were the happy days. Gone was my son's pleasant, happy life.

A few years prior to his breakdown, he started to show many troubling signs of emotional disturbances. He was not able to explain why he felt a particular way, or why he uttered certain statements. His behavior was difficult to manage. He refused to cooperate with the family. He was never happy. I kept wondering why my son is behaving in this rebellious manner. It was uncharacteristic of him to behave this way. He had always been an obedient child when he was growing up, now he is an out-of-control adolescent.

As time went on, a host of other symptoms began to emerge. He could no longer control his anger. He was very easily frustrated. He started missing classes. He stopped doing his chores.

At 16 years of age, while still attending school, he started working as a cashier in the fast food industry. He worked after school and on weekends. He took classes at a computer-training center and learned to use the computer. He was very proud that he typed 55 words per minute. That motivated him to seek employment with a temporary agency and he began working office jobs. It was difficult and challenging for him, but he attended school and continued to work.

A few months later, he received his driver license. He felt very proud when he saved enough money to buy his first car.

The pressures at school began to overwhelm him. He started to miss classes again, which caused me to contact the school for assistance. One morning the Principal visited us at home, and encouraged my son to continue attending school. However, he continued to miss classes and could not explain himself.

As time went on, his symptoms worsened. Eventually, he could no longer cope with high school. Before long, he dropped out. I was devastated. I encouraged him to return to school. I kept encouraging him not to give up. Soon afterwards, he was able to attend Alternative Education.

I was devastated when he dropped out of Alternative Education. I was worried sick about his future because he did not achieve his educational goals. He tried very hard to continue working. I kept encouraging him, not to give up and reassuring him that he would have a bright future because I knew he was struggling.

However, the symptoms continued. He started to miss work. Then, one morning he just would not get out of bed. He quit going to work all together, stayed in bed, and slept almost all the time.

His educational and career dreams vanished in front of my eyes. I was very heart broken at the thought that he must feel devastated at realizing that his life had fallen apart.

He then retreated from everyone and locked himself in his room. His bedroom became his haven. He was distraught, distressed, depressed and despondent. He was anxious and frustrated. It was extremely difficult to interact with him. He was angry, aggressive and restless. He was irrational and erratic.

His behaviors severely damaged his relationships with family and friends. And, the symptoms interfered with his ability to function.

During this entire time, my son never complained that he was feeling sick. He never discussed any of the symptoms with me. He just tried to be a brave young man.

As weeks turned into months, the symptoms intensified. He had a distorted perception of himself and of others. He did not care about anything or anyone. He did not have the abilities to admit or accept any personal successes or failures. His outlook for the future was pessimistic. The more he isolated himself the more he lost his self-esteem and self-confidence. He did not socialize with anyone.

As time went on, he became more hostile towards me and constantly screamed at me. There was constant tension and anger. His sleeping pattern became more erratic. One moment he was irrational and verbally abusive, the next moment he was remorseful.

In retrospect, I could see that my son was hallucinating, delusional and extremely paranoid. He had all the symptoms of schizophrenia.

The situation at home was grave. Many uncertainties hung over my head. Yet, after all those symptoms, I still did not know they were signs of the onset of schizophrenia.

The months leading up to his breakdown were filled with conflict, as he became more threatening towards me. One evening he became angry to the point that he took an egg from the refrigerator, threw it and hit me.

Since I did not know whether he would lose his self-control, I telephoned the police. By the time the police arrived, my son was calm, pleasant, and smiling as if nothing had happened. Still, I did not recognize that this kind of switching from calm to outrage, from fun loving to suicidal, were symptoms of schizophrenia.

One evening just after we finished dinner, my daughters went for a walk. Suddenly, one of my daughters ran into the house screaming that my son was sitting in the garage holding a kitchen knife. She looked frightened, and she was shaking. I wanted to run out to the garage to protect my son, tell him how much I loved him, and take the knife away from him. However, I stopped, realizing that perhaps that would not be the best approach.

I wasted no time. I immediately dialed 911. The operator told me not to go into the garage. She insisted that I stay on the phone with her.

She said that she had already dispatched the police and they would arrive in a few minutes.

Before the police arrived, my son re-entered the house with the knife and returned it to the kitchen. He was calm as if nothing had happened. Several police officers arrived a short time later. The police asked him why was he in the garage with a knife. He calmly responded, ***"I WAS JUST TRYING TO SCARE MY MOM."*** Shockingly, even then, I did not realize how serious the situation with the knife could have been.

By this time, the symptoms became relentless. Managing his life became impossible. He was in such anguish as well as inner turmoil, and when he was frustrated, He *yelled,* ***"I WOULD BE BETTER OFF DEAD!"***

When he continued talking about "**Not wanting to live,**" or that he did not, "**Ask to be born,**" I became very worried. It was only then that I really realized that this was not just mere teenage problems, or peculiar utterances, but signs of a serious mental illness.

Within weeks, my son had a complete mental breakdown and our lives were about to make an unexpected turn and instantly change.

In retrospect, I could see that my son was hallucinating, delusional and extremely paranoid. He had symptoms of schizophrenia!

Schizophrenia is one of the worst of all mental illnesses and I missed all the warning signs because I was very unaware of this illness!

I felt that I failed my son. I felt ashamed. I was heart-broken and had many regrets for years.

As a parent, I have had many regrets and have made many mistakes while raising my children. But, my biggest mistake was my **ignorance.** I truly thought those symptoms were just difficulties associated with teenage years, 'acting out,' as the experts say. I just thought his behaviors were unacceptable, not realizing that perhaps my son was experiencing psychosis. Unfortunately, they were much more than teenage difficulties. My son was, in fact, very chronically ill.

HOW IT PAINED MY HEART FOR MISSING ALL THOSE SYMPTOMS!

This difficult emerging situation would prepare me to cope with the tragedy that was yet to come.

There are countless warning signs. Becoming aware of them will ensure that mental illness is diagnosed early. The warning signs of mental illness include:

- Decreasing ability to function.
- Uttering of strange, disturbing comments.
- Acting out of character.
- Quitting school.
- Ceasing to work.
- Talking about violence, threatening comments, or talking about suicide or hurting someone.
- Isolating oneself from family and friends.
- Depression.
- Acting quickly.
- Lacking focus and concentration.
- Distorting reality.
- Moodiness.

- Failing to comply with instructions, and rules.
- Refusing to see a doctor or take medications.
- Manipulating everyone.
- Arguing.
- Forgetting, imaging and recalling imaginary details as information.
- Poorly executing instructions.
- Uncommunicative.
- Inability to reason or reflect.

Prior to my son's diagnosis and before he started taking medications, he had thoughts of suicide. Only at this point did I fully realize that he was having a serious mental breakdown.

Shortly after the incident with the knife, I scheduled an appointment for him to have an assessment. Unknown to me, the psychiatrist's office assigned an Intern to evaluate my son.

After a full hour, the Intern told me ***"Nothing is wrong with him."***

I explained to this Intern again all of the signs my son was experiencing.

He giggled, and said, **"I KNOW WHAT IT IS; THIS IS JUST a MOTHER–SON RELATIONSHIP, NOTHING IS WRONG WITH HIM."**

THE MOST DIFFICULT YEARS

The most difficult period of this illness spanned a 16-year period. My son was in turmoil. For almost all of those years, he refused to take his medication. And, for those 16 years, my family lived with doubts and fears. The challenges seemed insurmountable.

Law Enforcement
Countless times, when my son was experiencing psychosis, delusions and hallucinations, I needed help to take him to the hospital. For many days, I reminded him to take his medication, but he kept refusing. His health kept declining. I needed help from law enforcement.

Each time, I explained in detail **"My son is mentally ill, he is schizophrenic, he has refused to take his medication and that's why I need assistance to take him to the hospital."**

On one occasion, I dialed 911 for help. Within minutes, many police officers and two fire trucks responded. Instead of coming to my door, they parked on a side street. They were consulting with each other as to how to proceed.

On another occasion, similar to many other nights, my son could not sleep. I stayed up with him and we watched TV. A little past midnight, my son went outside for fresh air. After a few minutes, I heard heavy breathing and footsteps running up the stairs to my bedroom. I ran out of my bedroom to see what was happening. My son was trembling, and said, **"Mom, the cops are chasing me."** I was shocked. My son was watching TV with me for several hours. **"WHY IN THE WORLD WOULD THEY BE CHASING MY SON AT 1 AM?"** I screamed. I also started shaking. I ran down the stairs as quickly as I could. I ran to the front door and peered through the peephole. No one was there. I went to the window, moved back the blinds and peeped outside. I did not see anyone.

Suddenly, a flood of lights blinded me. Three police officers were hiding in the darkness. They ran to the windows still shining their bright lights on me. **"Open the door; we want to talk to you,"** They yelled to me. I opened the door, trying to cover my nightgown. **"What's wrong officer?"** I asked. **"Ma'am, tell your boyfriend to come out, we want to talk to him." "He is not my boyfriend, he is my son."** I replied. **"Get him out here, please,"** *they* *demanded.* I asked them why they wanted my son. They said they wanted to talk to him.

I later learned that, for several nights, they were staking out the house, looking for a *'suspicious person'.* A neighbor reported to the police that a *'suspicious person'* was standing outside on several nights. As it turned out, my son was that ***'suspicious person.'***

I explained to the two police officers that my son was suffering with schizophrenia and he had a great fear of police officers. They looked at each other. They did not know anything about schizophrenia. One of the officers tried to explain it to the other two officers. He told the other officer, **"It is similar to manic depression."**

Then they took my son outside and questioned him for about an hour.

Just then, a neighbor walked by and stopped briefly to say hello to us. The next day she told me that she heard and saw the whole incident. She was familiar with my son's illness and knew that he did not pose any danger to the neighborhood. She deliberately wanted the police to see that it was safe to walk outside at 1:00 a.m. in our community.

I **heavily** relied on the police for assistance because of my son's psychotic episodes. On one particular day, he had a relapse and was paranoid. The police responded to my phone call. When my son saw them, he became even more paranoid. He climbed through a bedroom window and up to the third floor of the building. They could not get him to come down. They called in a special team; they also could not convince my son to climb down from the roof.

Finally, they telephoned for a psychiatrist. The psychiatrist arrived and kept talking to my son who was still on top of the roof.

After a little while, my son calmly climbed down from the roof. As soon as his feet touched the ground, five officers jumped him, handcuffed him and transported him to the psychiatric hospital.

Three near Death Experiences

First Incident
This is what happened when two police officers startled my son. We had a horrifying, near death experience in my living room, in

front of me, that day. They almost blew my son's head to pieces.

On a beautiful, sunny Saturday morning, my son was fairly stabilized and feeling great. At around 11:30 a.m. that morning, my son asked my permission to go for a walk. I was thrilled that he felt well enough to take a walk. Thirty minutes had passed and he had not returned. I went out to the patio to await his return. Just then, a police car pulled up and stopped near the front of my house. My heart leapt as I watched two police officers exit their vehicle and stand by the vehicle with folded arms. I kept thinking, **"What Now."** After a few seconds, I asked the police officers if everything was ok. They replied, "*Everything is all right.*" I then let out a sigh of relief, thinking, "*Great, my son is ok.*"

Unknowingly, the worst HORRIFIC, BLOOD CHILLING, TRAUMATIC, UNEXPECTED EXPERIENCE OF MY LIFE was yet to come.

I remained on my patio waiting for my son. A few minutes later, I saw my son walking, very casually, towards the house. I was very happy to see that he was fine and was very happy to see him walking directly to the house. He slowly walked past the two officers. I was very proud of him because he did not seem paranoid of them.

Unknowingly, the worst was yet to come. The two officers followed him inside my house. They just walked right inside the house behind my son.

The police officers asked my son for the name and phone number of the boy he was walking with just moments earlier. My son did not answer the officers. Instead, he calmly walked straight up stairs. While he was upstairs, I explained to the officers that my son was suffering with schizophrenia and was very paranoid of police officers. I specifically wanted them to know that he was ill and that his behavior is not drug related, as some officers had previously believed.

After a few minutes, my son calmly came down stairs with a piece of paper in his hand. He handed the paper to one of the officers and continued walking towards the open front door.

As my son walked towards the open door, suddenly, to my surprise, one of the officers jumped in front of the door and blocked his exit. It startled me. It startled my son. What happened next turned into a nightmare, one that lasted for years.

My son was suffering with having paranoid schizophrenia. I told that to the police officers. I REPEATEDLY TOLD THE TWO POLICE OFFICERS THAT MY SON WAS PARANOID OF THEM AND THAT HE WOULD RUN. ONLY MOMENTS EARLIER, HE RAN WHEN HE SAW THEM. THAT IS WHY THE OFFICERS CAME AND PARKED AT MY FRONT DOOR. THEY KNEW HIS ADDRESS. THEY KNEW THAT HE RAN FROM THEM MANY TIMES PREVIOUSLY. Yet, they startled him by jumping and blocking him from exiting his home. He instantly reacted and struck the officer in his face. In an instant, they **slammed him onto the living room floor. They both jumped on him, handcuffed him, pepper sprayed him, and then put a gun to his head.**

I screamed at them not to kill him, that he was sick. My son lay on the floor defenseless and motionless. I kept screaming to the officers not to hurt him that he is paranoid.

I thanked God that they did not blow his head to pieces right there on my living room floor, right in front of me. They would have killed me too because I would not

have survived it. That scene will be forever etched in my mind as if it happened just yesterday!

He was a sick, paranoid, defenseless young man, much smaller than both officers. He was face down on the floor, in handcuffs, pepper sprayed and a gun at his head, yet, that treatment was not enough. The officers radioed to the police station for help. Even though I was a distressed mother begging them not to kill my son, and me, I kept thinking that they acted extremely cowardly.

Within minutes, six more officers arrived, including the Superintendent of Police. They dragged my son into the street. Seven of them formed a circle around him. They pulled down his pants. One of the officers pulled an object out of his pocket, and from where I was standing, **"They were assaulting my son with that object."** I continued screaming and attempted to go to my son.

As I tried to rush to my son to see what the police were doing to him, the seventh police officer blocked me from seeing what they were doing. I kept screaming **"HE IS SICK!"** Shockingly, the police said to me, **"If you interfere, we will lock you up."**

Whatever the police were doing to the backside of my son's body, *"That is between them and God."*

After they finished with what they were doing to him, they carried him to jail. That incident traumatized my son for many years.

Still, there were more horrific, traumatic experience occurred at the county jail.

Second Incident

The police kept him in the city jail for several hours, and then transported him to the county jail. I was frantic. His bail was set at ten thousand dollars. I could not afford to pay it. I went to the jail but I was not allowed to see my son.

Finally, after many days they told me he was in isolation.

I contacted the Public Defender's office.

For a full week or more, no one was allowed to see my son in jail. There were three court hearings. At each hearing, the Court ordered the Sheriff's office to release my son to the hospital. Each time, the Sheriff's office refused to comply with the Judges' orders.

After many failed attempts to see my son, I was convinced that he died in jail. The Public Defender's office sent two Attorneys to the jail to see my son. The jailers would not permit them to see him.

Finally, a private criminal attorney offered to help me. He went to the jail but they also denied him entry to see my son and they refused to explain themselves.

After quite a while, a person working at the jail in the medical section told me that they would transfer him to a psychiatric hospital. This went on for days. Although his jailers continuously gave me dates and times when he would be released to the psychiatric hospital, they never followed through. This ongoing delaying tactic caused me to be convinced, more than ever, that my son died in jail.

Finally, after many anguishing days, while I was talking to a nurse at the psychiatric hospital, she told me that the police had just arrived with my son. It was 3:00 a.m.

I was relieved. **HE WAS ALIVE!** I was very happy that he was not killed while in jail.

Early the next morning, I went to the hospital to see my son. He was in a very small, locked room. As I entered the room, he jumped off the bed and reached out to hug me. His first words *were, 'M-O-O-O-O-M.'*

I held him in my arms as I fought back my tears

He became very relieved when he saw me.

He was very thin and very sick. He appeared to be malnourished. His mental condition had significantly deteriorated from the morning when he went walking. It was extremely heart breaking that after I had diligently worked to stabilize my son, a walk on a beautiful, sunny morning could have caused such tremendous trauma at the hands of law enforcement officers. I stayed with my son and comforted him.

I wanted my son to tell me what the jailers did to him while he was in isolation, but he was in a paranoid state, and incoherent. He was paranoid that the police would lock him up, again.

I kept assuring him not to worry. I assured him that he would be safe in the hospital.

I stayed with him at the hospital for almost all of the day to comfort him.

During that time, he wanted to take a shower. When he removed his shirt, I saw open wounds on his back; the type that remains after a person has been beaten. He had many long open wounds on his entire back. I noticed that his feet also had cuts on them. Above his toes, were open holes; it looked as if a sharp object had pierced his flesh.

He did not want me to call the nurses to bandage his open wounds because he was paranoid that the police would lock him up again. I was very disheartened to see the cruel treatment that was inflicted on my son only because he was suffering with mentally ill.

I kept thinking, *"My mentally ill son is a human being. He wants to enjoy life as much as those who are not mentally ill."*

One day, a short time after his release from the hospital, a detective came to my house to arrest my son. By then I had sent him to another county for his protection.

It was during this time that many of his friends became intolerant of his mental illness. They called my son 'psycho' and 'stupid.' Soon, all telephone calls to him stopped.

Third Incident

A few years after my son's diagnosis, my neighbor's son became aware that my son was ill. He and his friends began to frequently laugh and mock my son because of his illness.

One day while his parents were at work, he had a party in the middle of the day. A large group of his friends attended. They invited my son, and he went. A little while later, they started to play heavy metal music. It was loud and pulsating. The music grew louder and louder until it was exploding. I was about to call the police, but just before I dialed 911, there was dead silence. The music stopped.

My gut feeling told me something was terribly wrong. I waited to see what would happen next.

After several minutes, I went back inside my house and my son followed. He walked towards me, and said, ***"M-O-O-O-M."*** Before he could finish saying the word 'mom,' he collapsed and fell to the floor. I screamed, ***"OH MY GOD.!" I rushed to his side; I held him and called his name. He did not respond. I immediately dialed 911.***

The Paramedics arrived but could not revive him. They rushed him to the emergency room. The doctors immediately pumped his stomach. The doctors told me that, **"He had five times the legal alcohol limit in his system."**

(Those young men all knew my son was ill. They should be ashamed of themselves for viciously treated a sick person in this way.)

I was uncontrollably shaking because I did not know if he would survive. There was enough alcohol in his system to have killed him if I had not been at home.

Support Group
Support Group meetings is not effective to someone with paranoid schizophrenia. my son.

Counseling Session
Counseling sessions did not help my son.

The Health Care System
My son received medical treatments from many different psychiatrists and hospitals. My experience with all of them evidenced one common practice: no compassion. *"They lacked the compassion I needed as a grieving mother.*

The American Health Insurance Portability, and Accountability Act of 1996 (HIPAA), prohibited medical personnel from discussing my son's health care with me without his consent because he was 18 years old. I should have obtained a Health Care Directive, but at that time, I was unaware that I would ever need such a document.

In California, the police escorted my son to the emergency room for treatments countless times. That was the only way to get him medical care as he was very non-compliant and could have been a danger to himself because he was hallucinating. In California, the Welfare and Institutions Code permits a police officer to involuntarily confine a person with a mental disorder that makes him or her a danger to self, or a danger to others, or if an individual is gravely disabled and cannot take care of himself/herself.

The Emergency Room doctors would then evaluate him/her then admit him/her to the psychiatric ward. Those visits are called "51/50 Hold."

The hospital could legally confine my son for 72-hours without his consent. If during, or after that period, his condition improved, the hospital will release him.

On the other hand, when his condition remained unchanged or worsened, the hospital kept him seven more days, without his consent. If his condition continued to deteriorate, and in many cases, it did, the hospital kept him for 14 more days, without his consent. After that period, he could ask to be released from the hospital, even if he is unstable. At this point, under the Institutions Code, the hospital is no longer allowed to prevent him from leaving the hospital.

On one occasion in California, a police escort was necessary to transport him to the hospital. After the initial three-day hold, my son was still hallucinating, yet the hospital released him, they put him into a cab, paid the cab fare and sent him home.

I was shocked when my son walked into the house without my knowledge!

I was upset that the hospital released him because my son was still hallucinating and needed to be in a safe place where he could not hurt himself or someone else. The hospital should have kept him until he was stable, or they should have called me, to drive him home since I was not just his mother but also his caregiver. However, the "Law" permits them to release a patient if the patient tells them him or her wants to leave.

That law is dangerous and irresponsible for someone who is experiencing delusions like my son.

Health Care Professionals
For over two decades, many health care professionals treated my son. During that entire period, no one has ever recommended a book, magazine, article or any other reading material that could have helped with the coping and recovery process.

Health Insurance
Health care is a basic human nccd. It is equally as necessary and important as food, clothing and shelter. No matter who we are, or our economic and social status, we all need health care. While many today are suffering from the lack of adequate mental health care, I am very appreciative that my son   received quality health care during much of the time that they were grappling with their mental illness.

Initially, my employers provided me with excellent mental health coverage.

Inadequate mental health insurance or the lack of mental health insurance is a very risky situation for society. Having adequate mental health insurance is crucial for the prevention of relapses, and suicide. Additionally, this ensures that they do not harm family or community members. During the untreated period of my son's illness, he frequently talked about "killing himself." Once he obtained the right medications and maintained his daily intake regimen, those feelings stopped. It is just good common sense for everyone to have access to mental health treatments.

Homes for the Disabled
If families need help to care for a loved one, there are places that accommodate them. They include "Group Homes," "Adult Care Homes," "Assisted Living Facilities," and "Board and Care Facilities." They all provide supervised, non-medical care for the disabled. They range from small facilities housing two to six individuals to large facilities, housing dozens of people. There are private and state funded homes. They must all adhere to strict guidelines.

Each state has its own set of rules. The Department of Social Services oversees the operation of these homes. If anyone has a complaint against any of these facilities, they can file it at any time with this department.

These facilities provide basic housing, and food, as well as distribute medications to the residents as prescribed by their doctors. Occupants are not patients; rather they are called, "Consumers," or "Residents."

The lack of housing for the mentally ill continues to be a national problem that is causing an increasingly chaotic and confusing situation for many individuals and families. This situation adds stress and anxiety to their lives. Since many who are chronically ill, especially those with severe schizophrenic symptoms, are unable to adequately care for themselves, and incapable of making housing arrangements for themselves. This is the reason that housing in private or state funded facilities is very necessary.

My experiences with my son's stays in board and care facilities were traumatic. They did not provide adequate, basic support services nor did they provide programs that were conducive to the healing or recovery process. I also found that the quality of care, and the type of workers at these facilities was deplorable.

My first encounter was when a hospital recommended a board and care facility. It was one of the worst experiences of my entire life.

My son spent one night in that facility. The next day, still very sick, still experiencing hallucinations and delusions, he walked approximately 15 miles to return home. There were many high-speed freeways between the hospital and home. I am still unsure as to how he managed such a dangerous journey.

I immediately telephoned the facility. The staff at that facility claimed that they did not even know that my son was gone for the entire day.

The next day I filed a complaint with the State Social Services Department.

Medication and Side Effects

Over the decades, several psychiatrists treated my son. They treated paranoid schizophrenia with a host of different medication. Most of them were ineffective for his condition. During his first psychotic breakdown, the hospital doctors initially treated him with the antipsychotic drug, Haldol. That was ineffective. His symptoms continued.

After several weeks, the doctors discontinued Haldol and began treating him with the drug, Elavil. My son continued to display all the symptoms, but to a lesser degree. After several weeks, they released him from the hospital, still in an unstable condition. Soon, that medication was also ineffective. Once again, his symptoms intensified and our lives spun out of control. He had to return to the hospital.

The hospital administered medication that lessened the symptoms and released him each time. His relapses and confinements to the psychiatric hospitals continued for many years. Over the years, he was confined to many different hospitals.

During the course of his illness, the doctors tried many other drugs including Prolixin. He responded to Prolixin along with Cogentin. Prolixin is used to control the symptoms and Cogentin for its side effects. Although he took Prolixin for many years, it did not successfully control all his symptoms. Before long, he was repeatedly hospitalized.

His illness continued to rage as the doctors tried many other types of medication such as Zyprexa, Risperdal, Abilify, Wellbutrin, Seroquel and Tramadol. His response to each of these was poor. His condition continued to deteriorate.

Risperdal helped him the most. But, once again, after taking Risperdal for a few years, he no longer responded to it.

HOPE SLOWLY DWINDLED YEAR AFTER YEAR

While he was taking extremely high doses of Seroquel, he developed type-2 diabetes. He is still taking diabetic medications to this day. He also developed an allergic reaction to the drug Tramadol.

For several years, he continued life in what his Psychiatrist described as a chronic, "gravely disabled state." he illness ravaged his life. Intermittently he enjoyed short periods of remission.

During the first sixteen years, along with countless confinements in psychiatric hospitals, there were also many month-long confinements in long-term care facilities.

There were many times when the family's strength to care for him waned. There were countless times when I needed a little time to reenergize. Those were the times when I had him admitted to board and care facilities. But, he never liked living in those facilities. He wanted to return home. He needed the love and security that his sisters and I provided for him and that was crucial to his recovery.

Many times, I compromised. I took him back home with us and hoped that the next day would be better. We were holding on to hope of stability, but **hope slowly dwindled year after year.**

Refused Medication

I respected my son's legal right to refuse medication. However, as his mother and primary caregiver, I could not sit by and let him suffer as he did, when I knew that medication would help him. I wanted to protect him and I wanted him to be safe and get well. I did everything in my power to get him the medical treatments that he needed and kept encouraging him to take the MEDICATION.

In my opinion and in the best interest of a mentally ill adult child, HIPAA Laws need to be reviewed and amended. I fought with all my strength to keep my adult son safe.

Relapses

My son had many, many hospital confinements and many relapses. One hospital recommended long-term confinement, which had to be approved by a judge. After his trial, the judge ruled in favor of a long-term care treatment plan. He was confined for several months. Even then, after his release, he continued to refuse medication and returned to his previous pattern of being in and out of hospitals.

With each relapse, our lives continued to be traumatic, filled with doubts, instability and upheaval. There were few indicators of the possibility of stabilization. However, even when there were apparent signs of improvements, another relapse occurred. After several of these experiences, I realized that improvement meant that relapse was imminent. My son's relapses were primarily because of not getting the proper medication and his non-compliance with post-treatment instructions, as well as other influences that disrupted his mental condition such as, his unshakable denial.

Caffeinated beverages, any kind of alcoholic beverages and sugar played a significant role in his relapses.

Severe stress -- such as a negative emotional state from social pressures or if he was planning a trip -- played a significant role in a relapse.

The relapses started with a gradual feeling of uselessness. He would gradually loose his self-esteem. He began to see his life as hopeless,

and he found no joy or purpose in living. He became increasingly negative about everything and everyone. He easily became agitated.

During these periods, there was never a minute of peace in the household. During those psychotic states, he jumped over walls, climbed on rails, climbed on roofs. On one occasion, he entered a neighbor's home by climbing through the window. Once, after discontinuing his medication, he relapsed, climbed to the top of a third floor building and jumped off. *"Thank God, he did not die."* He broke his ankle and spent weeks in an intensive care unit.

A typical relapse episode lasted anywhere from a few hours, to several weeks, and months, depending on the severity of the relapse. During this period, stress at home ranged from mundane to tragic when coping was near impossible.

His impairments were severe and detrimental. He had the necessary family and medical support as well as many opportunities to recover sooner, if only he had the mental capacity to make good decisions. Each relapse was accompanied by an insurmountable and incomparable amount of stress.

For years, his relapses and short periods of remission continued. After many frustrating years with no hope of recovery in sight, we left California and relocated to a small city in the beautiful Blue Ridge Mountains of Western North Carolina. I hoped that this change would be more conducive to their healing process.

During the first year living in the mountains, to my great disappointment, my son had another relapse and had to be hospitalized. Once again,

I was heartbroken. My hopes for stabilization were again shattered.

During his third relapse in that same year, while he was in the emergency room and awaiting approval to be admitted to the Psychiatric Ward, the hospital Psychiatrist refused to admit him, on the basis that his condition was too "***Chronic***," and that she did not want him as a patient.

A comment like this from a psychiatrist **was crushing because my family was suffering and in crisis**.

As the emergency room personnel frantically made telephone calls to the State Mental Institution, a friend recommended the Frye Regional Medical Center Psychiatric Ward in Hickory, North Carolina. The local hospital staff telephoned Frye Medical Center and they said they would admit him. Paramedics immediately transferred him to their facility. He was confined for several weeks.

After a careful examination of his medication history, the doctors at Frye Regional Medical decided to stop all his medication and they treated him with Clozapine (one of the oldest psychiatric medicines). This drug required strict blood test monitoring. He responded well for a while and we were hopeful. After a short time, our hopes diminished. The symptoms intensified.

His psychiatrist changed the medication to the name brand FazaClo, 700 mg per day, (a very large dose!). This medicine also requires strict blood test monitoring and manufacturer approval. Pharmacies are not allowed to dispense this drug without blood test results. At first, a weekly blood test was required for six consecutive months. After that, it had to be monitored every two weeks for another six consecutive months. After one year, it is required to be monitored on a monthly basis.

Finally, we were happy to have found medication that managed his symptoms! Yes, today, there is effective medication on the market that lessens the severity of mental illness. And we continue to live with the hope that there will be a cure someday soon.

His sisters and I were happy, that his condition dramatically improved. We were extremely overjoyed to see signs of recovery. That was six years ago, and the last time he was confined to a psychiatric hospital even though his manic state continued to be profound.

We had previously scheduled an appointment with a new psychiatrist. On the day of his appointment, my son was experiencing an extreme manic state. As soon as the psychiatrist saw him in that manic state, he immediately said, *"He needs to be on Lithium."* That decision would prove to be the greatest turning point in over thirteen years.

Finally, after years of devastations, he was correctly diagnosed – paranoid schizophrenia with type B-1 Bipolar. For thirteen years, all previous psychiatrists and psychiatric hospitals treated paranoid schizophrenia. They did not diagnose or treat the bipolar as a separate issue. Failure to accurately diagnose my son severely hindered his stability and progress. The psychiatrist decided to continue with the FazaClo; and immediately began treating the bipolar with 1000 mg of Lithium once a day. His diagnosis is now identified as Schizoaffective Disorder.

He has been taking both medications for six years and his progress has been phenomenal. About a year ago, with an effective diagnosis, along with our love and support, my son completely emerged from his denial, and assumed responsibility for managing his illness.

Although I tried many natural treatments, they did not help him. He responded well only to one prescribed medication, FazoClo, along with Lithium. When he tapered off, or stopped taking them, all manifestations of Schizophrenia returned. An aggressive medication regime is needed to avoid his return to the psychiatric ward, along with weeks and months of traumatizing the family.

Preparation and awareness were two key elements that helped me with preventing his relapses.

It was of paramount importance to me to have full confidence in my son's ability to heal. My confidence in his abilities strengthened him and made it easier for him to keep trying. He needed reassurance more than ever during this frightening time.

However, those challenges and obstacles were paving the way to coping, as more tragedies were yet to come. We would now be faced with the challenge of coping with the deaths of many loved ones.

Remissions

During remission, our lives returned to normal. It was a pleasant time in the family. My son felt a sense of belonging and felt good about himself. We enjoyed a 'normal' life. We engaged in fun activities and enjoyed each other's companionship. We laughed, and laughed and laughed. Throughout his entire ordeal, my son managed to retain his sense of humor. And, he sang and sang and sang. He sings songs when he is happy. He did daily chores such as preparing his meals, washing his dishes, shopping and doing his laundry. The days were stress free, anxiety free, and depression free.

HOW MY CHILDREN COPED

For the first 16 years my son could not cope with his illness.

How well my son copes with schizophrenia would depend on his own positive outlook of the future, and leaving his losses and all regrets behind him.

I began helping my son to cope with a sense of urgency. Since I didn't have any formal mental illness education or training, it was difficult to help him learn to cope. However, I was able to share with him *everything I learned* from research about schizophrenia. I also shared with him the knowledge I gained while caring for him as well as my accumulated years of working experiences.

I began training both my ill children by using *practical, common sense steps*, as follows:

SURPASSING LOVE: Like all children, my son flourished on my complete love and nurturing of them.

EMOTIONAL SUPPORT: They coped by accepting the emotional support I provided. I was by their side when they were fearful, when they were lonely or when they were just feeling sad. I comforted them. They needed to feel hopeful instead of experiencing feelings of failure and disappointment. I found ways to commend and encourage them.

CLEAR IDEA: I wanted them to have a clear idea of their illnesses and the skills I believed would help them to heal them fastest.

ACCEPTANCE: For the first several years, because of the *severity* of their illnesses, compounded with their complete denial of their mental illnesses, it was impossible for them to advance to the acceptance stage. I used the comparison between millions of people suffering from physical illnesses such as heart disease, stroke, cancer or diabetes, who must accept their illnesses, and the millions of others who are struggling with depression, stresses, or experiencing psychosis. Both groups must accept their illnesses before they will begin to heal.

BALANCE: I taught them how to have a balanced view of their illnesses and treat them the same as any other illnesses.

BELIEVE: I wanted desperately for them to believe that they would recover. Once they believed in themselves and trusted in their beliefs, they began walking down their pathways to recovery. First, they started coping. Then, they began advancing toward recovery.

ONE STEP: I encouraged them by telling them to take one small step at a time because each step was necessary for them to make small changes in their lives.

SMALL CHANGES: I taught them how to make small changes. They eventually understood that the only way to begin changing was by accepting their illnesses. After many years, they finally understood that no matter how small the changes in their thinking and lives were, those changes were vitally important to accepting their illnesses and helping them to cope.

HOPE: They quickly learned to embrace hope. They held on to the hope of recovery. They never gave up of hoping for recovery.

SHAME: In the beginning, they were ashamed to tell anyone that they were mentally ill. Over time, they were able to overcome their shame by realizing that there were no reasons to feel ashamed of their mental illness because it may suddenly strike anyone at any time.

HUMILIATED: At first, they felt humiliated by their mental illnesses. I engrained in them the fact that they did not need to feel ashamed. As the years passed, they ignored any feelings of humiliation and ignored anyone who tried to humiliate them.

SUFFERINGS: In time, they understood that they were not the only ones who are suffering, and that millions of others around the world were suffering from a form of mental illness. They also understood that those who are currently unaffected might someday succumb to mental illness.

FAULT: In the beginning, they felt that they might have caused their illnesses. Gratefully, they coped well when they understood that mental illness was not their fault, they did not cause it.

ANXIETY: They had periods when they suffered great anxieties, but I encouraged them to live by the scriptures encouragement not to worry about the future because tomorrow will have its own anxieties, problems, challenges and difficulties.

COURAGE: Happily, they did not allow the bitter effects of their illnesses to rob them of their courage to continue their lives.

NEVER GAVE UP: My children never gave up in their fight to survive their illnesses. They never gave in and never gave out either.

LOOKED BACK: I encouraged them to never look back on their past because there was nothing there to see. As a result, they seldom wondered what their lives might have been.

HOME ENVIRONMENT: They coped best when our home environment was supportive, compassionate and peaceful. They felt safe and unafraid.

GOOD DAYS: They distinguished their good days from their bad days. They appreciated and enjoyed the good days and did not waste time worrying about the other days when they were not feeling very well, or when their minds were deteriorating.

DISCERNMENT: They knew their limits and exited situations that could emotionally stress them.

REASSURANCE: When they felt depressed, I reassured them and reminded them, that their situation would improve.

FAILURES: They had many feelings of failure, but they learned to accept them and used them as motivational tools for their healing.

NEGATIVITY: They coped well when they ignored negativity. They recognized negativity in all its forms, extricated themselves from those situations and dwelled on positive thoughts and displaying positive traits. They also excelled when I did not accentuate their negative traits.

ENCOURAGEMENT: They thrived and coped well when others and I encouraged as well as reassured them with kind, comforting words. They felt refreshed.

APPRECIATE: When anyone showed genuine interest, offered sincere words of commendation or reassured them with a smile, they appreciated it.

KIND WORDS: Kind words from others were refreshing. They have power and they helped in the healing process.

PHONE CALLS: They appreciated any friends or relatives who called to check on them or to say hello.

VISITOR: They especially appreciated when anyone visited them.

SOCIAL: I taught them social skills. They visited friends and relatives who were kind, comforting, encouraging, understanding, positive, supportive and sympathetic. When friends greeted them warmly and with kind words, as well as listened to them, they progressed.

SUPPORT: They learned to accept any genuine offer of support from family and friends, and it was extremely refreshing when family and friends showed interest in them. In contrast, they avoided everyone who was critical and judgmental, including relatives who accused them of being 'lazy.'

RELAPSES: As time went on, they coped well when they understood how important it was to prevent any relapses, once they appreciated that frequent relapses significantly reduced their chances of recovery, they eagerly cooperated with the doctors' instructions and my retraining efforts.

PERSONAL SKILLS: They coped well when they developed personal skills for daily living with such activities as maintaining personal hygiene and etiquette.

HOME SKILLS: Years into their illnesses, as their health improved, they developed self-reliance skills such as performing light, household chores; doing their laundry; cleaning their rooms; washing their dishes; and preparing light meals.

ROUTINE: They had a daily routine such as taking the prescribed dosage of medication at the designated frequency.

MONEY SKILLS: Later, as they both progressed, they acquired advanced skills, such as money management. At first, although money had little value to them, I gave them an allowance to splurge on comfort food such as pizza, favorite smoothies and burgers.

I BEGAN TEACHING THEM TO REBUILD THEMSELVES BY DEVELOPING THEIR SKILLS AND TALENTS.

SELF: I helped them rebuild their self-worth and self-confidence to enable them to look forward to re-entering the workforce.

VISON: They coped by clearly envisioning what physical comforts they wanted and who they wanted to become.

FOCUS: They visualized their lives as completely free from illnesses. They did not focus on their illnesses. Instead, they focused on their talents, skills and abilities.

ADHERENCE: I was adamant about their strict adherence to medical appointments, and following prescribed instructions.

DECISIONS: They made independent decisions and learned appropriate, decisive self-expression.

THRIVE: They thrived when they knew that they were cared for, understood and appreciated regardless of their mentally challenged status.

OPTIMISM: In spite of all those struggles, my son displayed an incredible amount of zeal and optimism for their future life. As bleak as the outlook may have been, they were optimistic.

Obtaining and maintain their survival skills in the face of tragedies, is a reward to be viewed as strengths, not as weaknesses. They are also necessary tools for the day-to-day survival of mental illness.

VISUALIZED: They both visualized a positive, hopeful future.

POSITIVE: They remained positive throughout their journeys that they would learn to cope and that they would recover.

EMPOWERMENT: My children's lives were in total upheaval much of the time because of the changing tides of mental illness. Not just from day to day, but in many instances, from hour to hour. For them to cope, with any degree of success, meant that they had to *be constantly uplifted, and encouraged* as well as informed about any new treatments and medications. I empowered them by reading uplifting verses to them from the bible's book of Psalms and Proverbs. Their spirits were uplifted.

GOALS: After their symptoms decreased, I established goals. They were small goals that were reasonable and attainable.

PLAN OF ACTION: I continued to assist them in their plans for the future. I instituted a well thought out Plan of Action that included the furthering of their education, developing pre-job training skills, job search skills and work force participation skills.

SPIRITUALITY: Above all else, they consciously invested in their personal spiritual development as well as laid a faith-based foundation, which ensured that they developed the strength to successfully cope with their illnesses, accomplish their recovery goals and excel toward the futures of their choice.

THEIR OPTIMISM WAS BASED ON THE HOPE OF A POSITIVE, PROMISING FUTURE.

IMPORTANT COPING TIPS MY SON LEARNED DURING HIS JOURNEYS

☐ Never, ever look back.

☐ Take one day at a time; enjoy the good days and do not worry about the days that are disappointing or challenging.

☐ Display empathy and support toward each other.

☐ Learn long-suffering, kindness, and be self-sacrificing.

☐ Cling to hope.

☐ Find strength and courage.

☐ Be determined.

ACTIVITIES AND COPING

For the first several years, from 1991 to 1998, amidst my bleakest periods, from the beautiful coastlines of Southern California to the awesome Blue Ridge Mountains in North Carolina, we enjoyed many fun, simple activities that were free, but effective in helping the family to cope with the mental illnesses of two of its members. Besides prescribed medication, and my unconditional love, below is a list of the fun and simple activities that we enjoyed and that helped in the coping and recovery process:

☐ We took long walks and enjoyed the fresh air.

☐ We loved walking in the sunshine. We sun tanned to a golden brown along with our daily exercise.

☐ We enjoyed the fresh smell and the dramatic beauty of the flowers and blooming trees.

☐ Strolling around town on cool, breezy days was refreshing.

☐ Walks under beautiful moonlit skies and bright starry nights were very calming.

☐ We fed the birds and watched them, which filled us with a feeling of freedom.

☐ We walked on many nature trails and enjoyed the openness of the outdoors.

☐ We strolled around ponds and fed ducks.

❏We spent countless days relaxing in beautiful parks, enjoyed delicious picnic lunches and ate fresh berries and ripe watermelons.

❏We reclined in the lush, green grass and read, and studied the bible. Other times we just meditated.

❏We spent countless hours playing tennis and basketball.

❏We spent many hours walking on sandy beaches and enjoyed the cool ocean breeze. We watched the elegant surfers. We went looking for unusual seashells. We enjoyed many picnic lunches, enjoyed many bon fires on cool nights and ate marshmallows straight from the fire pits. We enjoyed sharing our food with the birds that always seemed hungry!

❏We enjoyed hiking up trails to the many wonderful waterfalls, and relaxed in the cool, refreshing waters of the Blue Ridge Mountains in Western North Carolina.

☐ We took leisurely, daily walks to the local library and read many books that really interested us.

☐ We enjoyed many relaxing walks on downtown Main Street, ate ice cream cones and enjoyed delicious pastries.

☐ We walked and window-shopped at local malls and enjoyed eating an egg roll or two.

☐ We listened to calming music such as beautiful religious melodies. We enjoyed listening to a wide variety of tranquility music.

☐ We swam at the pool, lounged under the sun or enjoyed a picnic lunch. Other times we just relaxed in the Jacuzzi.

☐ Exercise was important to us; and we frequently worked out at the gym.

☐ On weekends, we enjoyed friendly, home-based and park gatherings.

☐ We loved and enjoyed watching old movies.

☐ My daughter and I especially enjoyed massages and chiropractic treatments. Both helped to reduce our emotional pain and stress.

☐ My daughter and I spent countless hours in Lowe and Home Depot home gardening stores. We loved gardening. During the summer, we spent countless hours mowing the lawn and planted beautiful flowers.

☐ Many times, my son and I relaxed at fast food eateries such as Arby's, McDonalds, Burger King, Kentucky Fried Chicken, and we especially enjoyed Long John Silver from time to time. Since we were on a tight budget, we took advantage of buy one get one free coupons from mailings and occasionally from the back of grocery store receipts. These were fun times that afforded us the opportunity to build a strong relationship and a stronger bond with each other.

☐ One day, after my son visited the animal shelter and petted the animals, he saw a beautiful little kitten and he fell madly in love with it. He asked me if he could adopt the kitten. Against my better judgment, I said, "yes"; we went to the shelter and took the kitten home. Well, the kitten only lived with us for two weeks. It appeared that my son did not realize that work comes with having a pet!

☐ Continuous reinforcement of our family bonds by spending as much time as possible enjoying each other and developing their skills for the workforce.

STIGMAS TOWARD MY SON

Since the inception of mental illness into my children's lives over 22 years ago, my family has experienced many forms of stigmas. Yes, we have experienced stigmas from every sector of society. Some were subtle, while others were blatant.

The World Health Organization states, *"Stigma operates not only in the larger communities but also within the mental health service."*

My experiences with stigmas within the psychiatric field were profoundly disturbing.

(See Schizophrenia, Bipolar, Stress & Stigmas)

THE RECOVERY PROCESS

Traveling on his road to recovery was long, difficult and frustrating. At first, it was almost impossible to access that road. Continuing was even more difficult, as it was bumpy with twists and turns along steep, narrow, sudden curves that, if not skillfully navigated, would have most definitely resulted in plummeting into deep ravines from which there was no rescue.

Many times, giving up seem easier. In spite of the grimness and hopelessness of the situation, my son found paths to endurance and perseverance, which spurred him to continue his recovery journey.

There were numerous obstacles to his recovery. All along the way, there were obstacles. There were many periods of highs and lows; positives and negatives. There were smiles and laughter, as well as sadness and tears. We enjoyed many joyous times as well as much sadness. There were challenges, fears, stressors and depression. In light of these, we quickly realized that it would take a one day at a time approach to begin their recovery process.

How he viewed his life situation was central to his recovery process. For my son, the beginning of his recovery was when, for the first time, he was able to say the word, **"SCHIZO,"** with a smile on his face. I knew instantly that he was ready to begin recuperating.

My passion and drive for his recovery was foremost in my mind, and that propelled me to continue using my skills to encourage and support him.

Was recovery possible for my son?

ABSOLUTELY!

Yes, even though my son's recovery was slow compared to my daughter's, they both understood that the path to recovery was not the same for any two individuals. He experienced many severe relapses while my daughter recovered more quickly, with fewer relapses. Each progressed toward recovery at their own pace.

My son's last hospitalization was six years ago. Since then, he has been doing exceedingly well and for almost two years, with no signs of deterioration. Recovery is an on-going process for him.

Following, is a list of the attitudes that helped my son and daughter to begin recovering:

☐ *They both accepted their illnesses.*

☐ *They personally decided to begin their recovery journey.*

☐ *They were both ready and willing to make lifestyle changes that bridged to their specific roads to recovery.*

☐ *They both understood and accepted that, although there is no cure for mental illness, there is hope for living a quality life within the established economic system.*

☐ *They understood that the required journey required them to take one-step at a time.*

☐ *They understood that it could take years to achieve their recovery goals.*

☐ *They understood that they should never give up trying.*

☐ *They learned to be optimistic; to see hope where there was despair.*

☐ *They realized that there was an established relapse plan to ensure they would receive any necessary support to redirect them to their recovery paths.*

☐ *They realized that, as their primary supporter, caregiver and re-trainer, they could be confident that I would continue to tirelessly and unwaveringly monitor them for any signs of a relapse.*

Their healing process also involved taking his antipsychotic medications as scheduled and at the correct dosage, in addition to being the recipients of love, care, on-going support, respect, understanding and allowing him to make their recovery time-frame his own. These ingredients were the central components of his healing.

The recovery process was frustrating, but by taking one-step-at-a-time, he improved a little each day.

In the end, his personal interpretation of how he felt determined his recovery progress. He is the only one that can say with certainty that he has recovered.

Attitudes that helped my son and daughter in their healing process are as follows:

❑ They accepted their illnesses.

❑ They had a clear vision of recovery.

❑ They believed that their recoveries were possible.

❑ They had the desire to recover.

❑ They had a strong Will to work towards recovery.

❑ They stayed focused.

❑ They were positive.

❑ They received the proper medications and the correct dosages.

☐ They had unconditional extended family love, care, support, understanding and a strong nuclear-family support system.

☐ They knew their limitations and accepted them.

☐ They were persistent in finding ways to cope.

☐ They took one-step at a time.

☐ They looked at the bright side of life.

☐ They took a positive view of their illnesses.

☐ They had a positive view of the future.

☐ They found compassionate and supportive friends.

☐ They found neighbors who were encouraging and reassuring.

☐ They focused on what they could do instead of worrying about what they could not do.

☐ They kept their hope alive, and never wavered.

☐ They exercised regularly: walking, swimming and playing basketball.

☐ They had a stable routine: balanced diet and plenty of sleep.

☐ They engaged in regular, positive and worthwhile fun activities.

☐ They displayed strength, courage, determination, persistence and strength in the face of adversities.

☐ They had a daily household routine.

☐ They talked about their illnesses.

☐ They focused on developing healthy habits.

❑They read success stories about people recovering from mental illnesses.

❑They visited sick friends in their homes, the hospitals and nursing homes.

❑They encouraged friends who were discouraged.

These attitudes have been instrumental in helping my son to progress. By combining my training with these attitudes they developed the personal skills as well as job readiness skills that have resulted in my son living responsibly and independently as well as my daughter's enjoyment of her fulltime job and her optimism toward life.

HIS PROGRESS

At last, it is thrilling, that after 22 years, my son is finally out of denial and on his road to self-reliance.

He has been developing his job readiness skills and is now leading a meaningful and independent life. He is also working diligently at adjusting his lifestyle to include foods, activities and associates that are conducive to becoming a healthier person.

For years, my son remained in denial. He refused to accept or understand his illness. Additionally, he was oblivious to developing the proper views or motives toward recovery. Today, he has accepted responsibility for managing his illness and creating the life that he wants to live. NO MORE DENIAL!

For decades, my son was ashamed of his mental illness. When asked by doctors what he thinks is wrong with him, he would always say, *"I just feel a little depressed."* Today, he speaks openly with his doctor. He is no longer ashamed of his illnesses.

For two decades after his adolescence, my son lived with me and at times in and out of

Assisted Living Facilities. Today, he is living responsibly and independently.

For decades, he showed no signs of reasonableness. Today, he is reasonable.

For years, he could not make decisions, no matter how small. Today, he is making wise decisions. He is now capable of handling any situation with thoughtfulness and maturity.

On August 8, 2012, two decades after my son became ill; he expressed his interest in reading success stories about others who are recovering from schizophrenia. A week later, as I was reading the local newspaper, he asked to read the sports section of the paper. *One can only imagine the joy and happiness I felt.*

For the first 16 years, my son fought against taking his medications. Today, he manages his own medication, schedules and independently maintains his doctor's appointments with his psychiatrist and primary care physicians.

Today, he is studying the self-help guidebooks and training guides that I wrote to help him reintegrate and prepare to overcome the challenges daily life and of job searching.

Periodically, he also takes classes at the local community college.

The most significant achievement of my son's recovery process was his acceptance of responsibility for managing his mental health care. My greatest joy is sharing in his experience of unparalleled success to the point that I can safely use the term, "recovering." I am convinced that it was -- and continues to be -- his self-commitment, desire for well-being and overall optimism that, combined with my devotion and practical skills development training, has resulted in his recovery.

22 years ago, my son's prognosis was, *"He may never recover."* The family felt hopeless at that time. Today, we are all enjoying seeing him on his road to recovery.

I applaud my son for all his efforts. His progress surpasses my expectations. I am amazed at how well he is progressing.

The resiliency he displayed is **OUTSTANDING**! His progress to date is **REMARKABLE**!

Today, I am inspired to share my journey with everyone.

Today, I know that managing schizophrenia and being a contributing member of society is possible.

Today, I am inspired to share my coping and recovery empowerment methods and job training skills with others who want to access their path to recovery.

What inspired me to share this story is the success my sons have had in overcoming the adversities that resulted from schizophrenia. Yes, when my son lost decades of his life to this chronic mental illness, he became isolated and fearful, and lost his abilities to continue with his life. His abilities to continue with relationships were gone. Even the thought of education and job training goals or of a job search process tremendously stressed him. In the end, my son is alive and happy today because I devoted all my time, energy and resources to caring for him.

CONCLUSION

Parents all over America living in households and communities that create modern day stressors should be concerned and worried about their children's mental health, keeping in mind that stress is an inducer of mental illness, especially if there are genetic predispositions to this neurological imbalance.

The reason for concern is that anyone's son or daughter, brother or sister, mother or father, friend acquaintance or neighbor could at any time succumbed to a neurological imbalance induced by daily stressors. It shatters lives and may take years to stabilize or result in never being able to return to a quality of life conducive to community living.

Coping is difficult. Accessing the road to recovery is even harder. To cope with mental illnesses, many may turn to illegal drugs, alcohol, or promiscuity in desperation to escape their feelings of bewilderment about what is happening to them.

Most may have feelings of hopelessness, uncertainty and despair. Many family relationships are broken, and marriages may fail. Too many may even turn to violence and crime, and instead of receiving the therapies and medication that they need, become housed in an already overcrowded and financially overburdened prison system. The most unfortunate, who cannot cope, MAY COMMIT SUICIDE OR MURDER.

AMERICANS HAVE THE POWER TO CHANGE THESE OUTCOMES!

Studies have shown that mental illnesses lead to unemployment; homelessness; poverty; overcrowded street corners, parks; jails and prison systems; and increase overall criminal activity including white-collar crime, and violence in all its forms which is perpetrated onto healthy members of society in the form of domestic abuse, sexual harassment, sexual trafficking and child exploitation. If a person does not have access to the proper medical attention, left undiagnosed and untreated, a person will become despondent, and ultimately, may take his or her life, or endanger someone else's life. This is PROFOUNDLY DANGEROUS to a civil society and will result in its destruction one person at a time, one household at a time, one community at a time.

Thousands of the mentally ill are homeless. Studies have shown that, "At any given time, there are many more Americans with untreated severe psychiatric illnesses living on America's streets than are receiving care in hospitals. Americans with untreated schizophrenia and manic-depressive illness comprise one-third or 250,000, of the estimated 744,000 homeless population. The quality of life for these individuals is abysmal. Many are victimized regularly.

It has been stated that women with schizophrenia and bi-polar disorders are more likely to be raped multiple times.

It has been stated that adequate mental health care is lacking in ALL American cities. It continues to be a problem, and is associated with high levels of social burden and costs leading to municipal financial failure, as well as an incalculable amount of individual pain and suffering.

Today, the mental health sector is making significant progress in raising awareness about early diagnosis and treatment options. However, until there is a cure, Americans will continue to suffer.

What is America's mental health outlook?

Empowering each person to become responsible for maintaining his or her mental wellness or accessing mental health care is a very feasible and cost effective plan.

Each America has the power to alleviate the mental suffering of another America by caring for his or her mentally ill loved ones. They can encourage non-stigmatizing access to mental health providers and ensuring the availability of re-training options for those who have begun their journeys toward recovery with the expectation of experiencing their return to a healthier quality of life as a responsible, contributing member of society.

Notes

❑ *Schizophrenia is a complex disease of the brain, and a genetic disorder.*

❑ *It is not contagious.*

❑ *It is not caused from bad parenting, childhood traumas, average daily stresses, or from any financial hardships.*

❑ *Excessive amounts of stresses can trigger this illness.*

❑ *It is not anyone's fault, not mine, not yours, not anybody's.*

❑ *Although it may appear to look like a split personality disorder, it is not.*

❑ *Although science has made great progress, there is no cure.*

❑ *It is treatable and manageable.*

❑ *The brain, like other organs in the body, can get sick, and it can get well.*

❏ *Psychosis is a state of mental impairment. It distorts one's perceptions of everything.*

❏ *Hallucinations are caused by disturbances in sensory perception and the inability to separate real from unreal experiences.*

Group Homes

"Group Homes," "Assisted Living Facility," and "Board and Care Facility," all provide supervised, non-medical care for the disabled. Some are small, housing two to six people, while others are large houses and can accommodate dozens of residents. Some homes are privately own while others are state funded. They all fall under strict guidelines. Each State has its own set of rules. The Department of Social Services oversees the operations of these homes. If anyone has complaints against one of these facilities, they can file it with this department at any time. If your loved ones do not need hospital or nursing home medical care, and you need help in caring for them, there are places that can accommodate them. These facilities provide basic housing, food, and administer medications as prescribed by the doctors. Occupants are not patients; rather they are "Consumers," or "Residents."

Housing

As housing continues to be a national problem for the mentally ill, more and more people -- families and the mentally challenged -- are left in chaos and confusion, and with added stress and anxiety. Ensuring access to facilities that are staffed with those who have received proper training is crucial since many chronically ill Americans, especially those with schizophrenic symptoms, cannot adequately care for themselves, and families providing primary care usually need time to refresh themselves from the trauma of managing a loved one's illness. Those who are mentally ill are usually incapable of making housing arrangements for themselves, which is one reason that they may need housing in those facilities.

Depression

Depression or depressive disorders, is a leading cause of disability in the United States as well as worldwide. It affects an estimated 9.5 percent of American adults in a given year. Nearly twice as many women as men have depression. Epidemiological studies have reported that up to 2.5 percent of children and 8.3 percent of adolescents in the United States suffer from depression.

HIPAA

The American Health Insurance Portability and Accountability Act of 1996. (This Act is dangerous. It brings much heartaches to families caring for the ill. It needs to be amended to allow loved ones to make health care decisions for the mentally impaired relative.

A 51/50 Hold

This means that when a patient is brought to the Emergency Room by the police, the psychiatric hospital can legally confine that person for up to 72-hours without the person's consent.

The Law of Thirds:

"Statistically, one third of all diagnosed will recover completely, one third will improve over time and one third will not improve." This is based on J. H. Stephens' summary of 25 studies of 44,000 patients, followed on the average for 10 years, and is a commonly held ("Rule of Thirds" coined by American Psychiatrists.)

Quotations

The National Mental Health Association stated, *"Mental health problems affect one in every five young people at any given time. An estimated two-thirds of all young people with mental health problems are not receiving the help they need."* The article further states, *"Suicide is the third leading cause of death for 15- to 24-years-olds and the sixth leading cause of death for 5- to 15-year-olds."*

Worldwide in 2014, more than 400 million people suffer from depression, 24 million suffer from schizophrenia, and 60 million suffer from bipolar disorders. Many millions more suffer from some form of mental disorders or mental problems. (WHO October 2014.)

World Health Organization issued a Release stating, *"There are nearly 80 million people around the world with severe mental disorders, such as schizophrenia and bipolar affective disorder (manic depressive illness). In addition, 400 million people suffer from depression, millions more are undiagnosed and untreated."*

According to Dr. Cheryl Lane, PhD. www.schizophrenia.com, *"Attempting to find new work after a diagnosis of schizophrenia can be particularly difficult. If a potential employer is aware of the person's diagnosis, discrimination may hinder landing a job. Also, significant stigma is associated with any major mental illness."*

Dr. Lane further states, *"A possible solution for many individuals is to become involved in some sort of vocational training or rehabilitation program. They can learn new skills and get help with learning or improving social skills. These programs can also help them function more fully and develop better thinking skills. Additionally, working with a psychotherapist can help with self-esteem issues, stress management and making the best choices in terms of whether to work."*

Columbia University's Department of Psychiatry stated that *"To understand and promote recovery from serious mental illnesses, it is important to study the perspectives of individuals who are coping with mental health problems. The aim of the present study was to examine identity-related themes in published self-narratives of family members and individuals with serious mental illness. It adds* *to the body of research addressing how identity affects the process of recovery and identifies potential opportunities for using published narratives to support individuals as they move toward positive identities that facilitate recovery."*

The National Institute of Mental Health (NIMH), stated, *"Schizophrenia is a chronic, severe, and disabling brain disorder that has affected people throughout history. About 1-2 percent of Americans have the disease."*

World Fellowship for Schizophrenia and Allied Disorders, states, *"Schizophrenia is the most persistent and disabling of the major mental illness...While it is treatable in many cases there is yet no cure..."*

A psychiatrist, as recorded in a medical journal [16 (2) 2003], was quoted as saying, *"It is well known that schizophrenia is a chronic, generally life-long, mental illness that significantly debilitates afflicted individuals and severely compromises their function and quality of life."*

The Nutritional Management of Schizophrenia described schizophrenia in this way, *"Schizophrenia may be caused by* *genetic predisposing factors or environmental influences."*

University of Alberta Press Release, stated, *"Schizophrenia is a biochemical brain disorder characterized by delusions, disordered, thinking, hallucinations and a lack of motivation and energy."*

U.S. National Institutes of Mental Health (NIMH) stated, *"1.1 percent of the U.S. population age 18 and older in any given year."* *The article goes on to state, "Scientists have long known that Schizophrenia runs in families, it occurs in 10% of people who have first-degree relatives with the disorder." Additionally, it stated, "Many people with Schizophrenia improve enough to lead independent, satisfying lives."*

National Alliance on Mental Illness stated, *"Schizophrenia is a serious mental illness that affects 2.4 million American adults over the age of 18."*

The American Psychiatric Association stated regarding one possible cause of Schizophrenia, *"Although the origin of Schizophrenia has not been identified, Scientists know that there are some hereditary or genetic* *predispositions for the disease because it runs in families."*

American Psychiatric Association, Jeffrey Draine, Ph.D. and several or his colleagues wrote an article stated, *"With an improved understanding of the disease and effective therapies, those with schizophrenia can have a full life, hold a job, and live in the community or with their family."*

World Health Organization stated, *"More than 90% of all cases of suicide are associated with mental disorders such as depression, schizophrenia, and alcoholism,"* notes Dr. Benedetto Saraceno, Director of the Department of Mental Health for WHO, October 9, 2006.

The National Advisory Mental Health Council of the WHO stated, *"Schizophrenia is a (mental) disorder associated with high levels of social burden and cost, as well as an incalculable amount of individual pain and suffering."*

World Health Organization, *i*n a 1992 article, *quoted Leete as saying, "Stigma is shameful and displays a shameful part in human behavior.*

Stigma is damaging and destructive, it is a multi-layered and complex problem."

WHO published an article by Deegan *in 1980. The article stated, "Stigmas act as a powerful barrier to treatment not because of the fear of being labeled as mentally ill, but because too often mental health professionals and mental health services as a whole, often in a subtle way display negative or rejecting attitudes towards users and perpetuate practices fostering segregation, dependency and powerlessness.*

The Queensland Alliance for Mental Health observed, "P*eople with mental health problems are "frequently the object of ridicule or derision and are depicted within the media as being violent, impulsive and incompetent." It also found that the myth surrounding violence has not been dispelled, despite evidence to the contrary.*

Mental Illness Policy stated, *Americans with untreated schizophrenia and manic-depressive illness comprise one-third or 250,000, of the estimated 744,000 homeless population. The quality of life for these individuals is abysmal. Many are victimized regularly.* (mentalillnesspolicy.org)

Social Psychiatry and Psychiatric, in a 1994 study stated, *"Women with schizophrenia and bi-polar disorders are more likely to be raped multiple times."*

Regarding recovery, the American Psychiatric Association said, *"With an improved understanding of the disease and effective therapies, those with schizophrenia can have a full life, hold a job, and live in the community or with their family,"*

"More than 90% of all cases of suicide are associated with mental disorders such as depression, schizophrenia, and alcoholism," notes Dr. Benedetto Saraceno, Director of the Department of Mental Health for WHO.

Resources

American Psychiatric Association
1000 Wilson Blvd, Suite 1825
Arlington, VA 22209-3901
Phone Number: (703) 907-7300
Email Address: apa@psych.org
www.psych.org

World Health Organization
www.who.org

Author

Alyse King is the mother of four courageous children, one wonderful son and three delightful daughters. She is also a grandmother of one beautiful granddaughter and four adorable grandsons.

For over two decades, Ms. King has tirelessly focused her attention on caring for two of her four children who had been struggling with chronic illnesses since they were teenagers. She has successfully helped them cope with their illnesses and reintegrate into society by retraining them to live independently and become financially self-reliant, provided them with the soft skills training that are vitally important to self-improvement and skills for the job market.

Ms. King's happiness about her ability to help her son and daughter has encouraged her to share the "recovery techniques" she used. She self-published seven books titled, "A Letter to Schizophrenia from a Mother," "Schizophrenia- Coping," "When Bi-Polar Strikes," "140 Ways Coping with Depression," "Schizophrenia, Bi-Polar, Stress and Stigmas," "Finding Hope in a Hopeless World," and a self-help Workbook titled, "Day After Day Coping with Mental Illness - Support for Individuals and Families."

These books tell how she rebuilt her children's lives by helping them with skills that are necessary for coping, managing daily in-home routines, adhering to medical reminders, as well as the increasing joy she felt after each hurdle that marked their movement beyond illness.

The experiences gained as the mother of children who are successfully recovering from illnesses, as well as being their full time caregiver, instructor and re-trainer, has enabled her to accumulate many years of expertise. Additionally, her prior experience as a trainer in the private sector has added necessary, unique tools for writing these books.

Alyse King also self-published three Self-Help Guides titled, "Reintegrating after Traumatic Life Experience for: "Self Improvement," "Job Preparation," and "How to Keep Your Job." The Workbooks provide continuing education and training for returning to employment or becoming financially independent. The Workbooks share the systematic techniques that Ms. King used in helping her children to develop personal skills and skills for hunting for a job, securing the job and holding the job.

She also self-published, "A Trainers' Manual for "Self-Improvement, Job Preparation, Job Retention." The Trainers' Manual provides guidance to all who wish to develop programs to help others to find work or achieve financial independence.

Alyse also self-published, "Comfort and Hope – Death-Reflections from Scriptures," and three non-fiction titles, "A 30-Day Online Romance, Based on a True Story - Part 1," "Confessions from A 30-Day Online Romance, Based on a True Story - Part 2, and "A

Follow-Up of Confessions from A 30-Day Online Romance, Based on a True Story - Part 3."

Ms. King grew up and was educated on a beautiful Caribbean Island; married in her 20's and has been a homemaker, mother and sole provider for her family. Later, divorced, she relocated to Southern California with her four children.

The author currently resides in the beautiful Blue Ridge Mountains in Western North Carolina. Her son and youngest daughter also live in North Carolina. Her other two eldest daughters and all five grandchildren remain in Southern California. She frequently travels to California to visit her family and friends.

Ms. King's goal is to utilize her expertise in both the health and educational sectors. For the past several years, she has been working towards that goal by volunteering her time to help friends who are struggling to cope with mental illness.

Website: cmitrainingservices.com
E-mail: cmitrainingservices@gmail.com
http://www.amazon.com/-/e/B001KE71BQ
https://www.smashwords.com/books/search?query=alyse+king
http://www.linkedin.com/in/alyseking
https://www.facebook.com/alyse.king.12382

https://www.youtube.com/watch?v=S0OHV_5213Y

NOTES

NOTES

NOTES